DAILY YOGA JOURNAL &
GRATITUDE NOTEBOOK

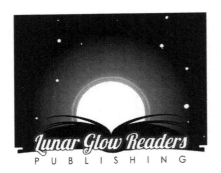

Cover and page design by Cool Journals Studios - Copyright 2016

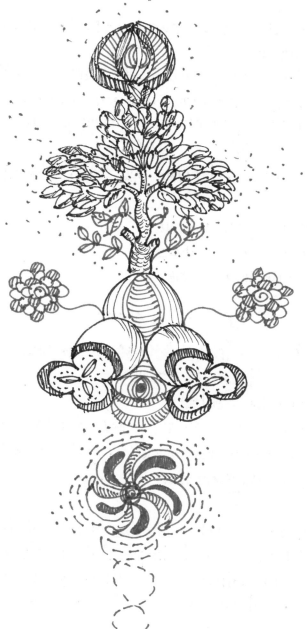

DUŠICA BAJIĆ
2017/18 Yoga Journal

INHALE. EXHALE. REPEAT.

MON
9/11/2017
'Our every single moment is precious & valuable'
#Adyashanti
Fairytale story telling at bedtime with Darling
Mook! ❤️ #princessandthegreenpea
#being in the flow of life #being present

☐ AM YOGA ☐ PM YOGA ☒ MEDITATION **IN ACTION**

TUE
9/12/2017 — Meeting with Sean Deoni

☑ Being Spontaneous
☑ Taking a chance
☑ Being in a Flow

☐ AM YOGA ☐ PM YOGA ☒ MEDITATION **IN ACTION**

WED
09/13/2017 ADYA SANGA — Live web event
(PEACE ROOM)
MFA evening with Seetal
"I've learned that people will forget what you said,
people will forget what you did, but people will never
forget how you made them feel."

☐ AM YOGA ☐ PM YOGA ☒ MEDITATION

THU
Peel, Peel, Peel (like the onion) all the layers
of unconscious beliefs that are blocking the
full manifestation & expression of your true
being. #truth #peace #grace #compassion
#love
DAY #2 PRACTICE with Meghan: Act of Self Love

☒ AM YOGA ☐ PM YOGA ☐ MEDITATION

INHALE.EXHALE.REPEAT.

9/15/2017 **FRI**

MFA - Moore
MFA - Dinner with Rosie

☐ AM YOGA　☐ PM YOGA　☐ MEDITATION

9/16/2017 **SAT**

Basho - lunch with Chandler + Samuel
Yogaworks BackBay - Jason Crandell (SPLITS)
Dinner with Louise in Somerville
Rupert Spira U-tube (basic & Foot - illustrator of Ego)

☐ AM YOGA　▨ PM YOGA　▨ MEDITATION

9/17/17 **SUN**

Car Ride to NYC
100,000 BUDHAS - YOGA (ABC Home, 888 Broadway)
with AMANDA, DJ DREZ, & MC JOSI

Heart Opening
Love
Tears
Truth

☐ AM YOGA　▨ PM YOGA　▨ MEDITATION

❧ THINGS MOST GRATEFUL FOR THIS WEEK ❧　GRATITUDE

1. Fortitude in blessed Life
2. Opportunities for Creative work
3. Freedom to explore the World
4. Lack of Fear & presence of LOVE
5. ABUNDANCE
6. Ability to take Care of others ❧

INHALE. EXHALE. REPEAT.

MON

9/18/2017   6-7PM Meditation with Rich Ray
Inquiry into Awareness practice.

☐ AM YOGA   ☐ PM YOGA   ☒ MEDITATION

TUE

9/19/2017
CODY Application: Shoulder's Picante by Megh → Instead I did: Legs PICANTE
Meditation: 10 min a Lecture with Echart Tolle
* Every challenge can be met in → Doing way
                                    → ~~being way~~
"The BALANCE OF BEING & DOING" → Best in doing Both
                            (TRANSENDENCE)
☐ AM YOGA   ☒ PM YOGA   ☒ MEDITATION   Accept completely anything
                                        (condition) that you experi

WED

Any Challenge is a great blessing.
~~Every lifetime~~ evolves through Challenges.

MFA: Mark Rothko
MFA: French Movie
~~READING~~
☐ AM YOGA   ☐ PM YOGA   ☐ MEDITATION

THU

AM: Meghan Currie - Spoonfulls
PM: Yin with Patric   Henry James
"I am sure you've an excellent spirit; but don't try to bear
more things than you need." "Hard things have come to you
in youth, but you mustn't think life will be for you all
Hard things. You've the Right to be Happy. You must
☒ AM YOGA   ☒ PM YOGA   ☒ MEDITATION/Spiritual Lecture: Echart Tolle
make up your mind to it. You must accept any form in which
happiness may come.

INHALE. EXHALE. REPEAT.

9/22/17

IN alignment - what is
take action from a peaceful place!
ACTION with a loving way / manner.

AM → OR
After work / baby MRI

(conditioned anything is at the surface of ego-driven individuals)

BEING & DOING
(Realise the (being) aspect of being → otherwise fruitless life
(Goete : No great piece of work has been created in luxury)
What ever happens: Be where you are!
Spacious Moment of No thought!

☐ AM YOGA   ☐ PM YOGA   ☐ MEDITATION   **ALERT PRESENCE!**
(without calling any words or thoughts)

9/23/17

Wacthau Call
Satsang with Peter
(3-5 PM)

Movies @ Home
Max

☐ AM YOGA   ☐ PM YOGA   ☒ MEDITATION

Mooji @ the Gas Pump II
(1:48)   WHAT AM I ?
Next step is to: 9/24/17
* KNOW this so completely, that you
STOP KNOWING IT.
Recognition & Realization deep in your
Heart ... the actions & pursuits will come naturally
Deeply abide in consciousness
You will know what is next   Next is simply what   comes w/o being
Next breath just follows.   Concerned!
spontaneity of actions.

(Be entwined with your true Nature)

☐ AM YOGA   ☒ PM YOGA   ☒ MEDITATION

1:55 All of Life is an extraordinary   spectacular
THINGS MOST GRATEFUL FOR THIS WEEK   tremendously
Life is not what you   wonderful   beautiful.
think it is a Life is   mistical experience!
becomes exactly
what you think
it is   • Life as if you have no rights
(Like you have no entitlement)

4. Love
5. Family   Whatever is happening is a path
to enlightenment!
6. Abundance   random happenings - all perfect

Health
Vitality   Beauty in the world

INHALE.EXHALE.REPEAT.

9/25/17
MON

NIRODAH = stillness

True nature of the self within a is the steady state in the face of any difficulties that may arise!

☐ AM YOGA ☐ PM YOGA ☐ MEDITATION

9/26/17
TUE

You suddenly realize that you are not your body, your thoughts, your job, your home.

You have a calm sanctuary (inner sanctuary) that is the root of your true sense of self. You see yourself through the eyes of Spirit.

☐ AM YOGA ☐ PM YOGA ☐ MEDITATION

9/27/17
WED

Stillness is your access point to this inner world!

KINO YOGA

☐ AM YOGA ☐ PM YOGA ☐ MEDITATION

9/28/17
THU

MFA - Ballett with Rosie

☐ AM YOGA ☐ PM YOGA ☒ MEDITATION

INHALE. EXHALE. REPEAT.

9/29/17
FRI

9AM Yoga 10min

11-8 PM OR Shift
8:00 PM Baby Brain PERL

▨ AM YOGA ☐ PM YOGA ☐ MEDITATION

9/30/17
SAT

→Michelangelo Moue @ MFA 11:00AM (Stayed in Bed)
Beogradsko pozorište 6 PM

Home Yoga 10min
▨ AM YOGA ☐ PM YOGA ☐ MEDITATION

10/81/17
SUN

Exhale - Yoga Twist/Abs
Exhale - Deep tissue with Jash →Michael

▨ AM YOGA ☐ PM YOGA ▨ MEDITATION

THINGS MOST GRATEFUL FOR THIS WEEK

GRATITUDE

1. Being Healthy & Calm
2. Having a Wonderful Family
3. Feeling Love & Compassion
4. Being at Peace
5. Making a Change in other people's lives
6. Having a Wonderful Life (manifestation of deep dreams & wishes

INHALE.EXHALE.REPEAT.

10/2 MON

Yin Yoga (Meghan Currie Chest Openers)

☐ AM YOGA ☒ PM YOGA ☒ MEDITATION

10/3 TUE

(Meghan Currie - Shoulders Picante)

☒ AM YOGA ☐ PM YOGA ☒ MEDITATION

10/4 WED

Grand Rounds with J. Neurosci editor

FULL MOON

☐ AM YOGA ☐ PM YOGA ☐ MEDITATION

10/5 THU

☐ AM YOGA ☐ PM YOGA ☐ MEDITATION

INHALE.EXHALE.REPEAT.

CR

10/6
FRI

Packing

☐ AM YOGA ☐ PM YOGA ▨ MEDITATION

10/7
SAT

Travel to Phoenix, AZ

Lunch @ SPA.

menu
white beans
kale, red onion } salad
Salmon   with

☐ AM YOGA ☐ PM YOGA ▨ MEDITATION

Yoga - Meghan Cleere - lesson 1

10/8
SUN

▨ AM YOGA ☐ PM YOGA ☐ MEDITATION

THINGS MOST GRATEFUL FOR THIS WEEK

GRATI
TUDE

1.
2.
3.
4.
5.
6.

10/9 MON	Meghan Currie - Lesson 2

☑ AM YOGA ☐ PM YOGA ☐ MEDITATION

10/10 TUE	Meeting with Peter Cutler

Sedona, AZ

GODDESS

☐ AM YOGA ☐ PM YOGA ☐ MEDITATION

10/11 WED	Meghan Currie - lesson 3

☑ AM YOGA ☐ PM YOGA ☐ MEDITATION

10/12 THU	DRIVE TO Sedona

ENCHANTMENT
* Mii amo VORTEX *

☐ AM YOGA ☐ PM YOGA ☑ MEDITATION

INHALE. EXHALE. REPEAT.

5:15AM → 8:30AM → Submitted RO3
Cathedral Rock Climb

Pink Jeep Tour

☐ AM YOGA   ☐ PM YOGA   ☐ MEDITATION

Church Rock Vortex
Mii Amo Spa
Como - Social Massage c̄ RoseMarie ♥

Boston Canyon Track

☐ AM YOGA   ☐ PM YOGA   ☐ MEDITATION

Sedona

Phoenix

Boston

☐ AM YOGA   ☐ PM YOGA   ▨ MEDITATION

THINGS MOST GRATEFUL FOR THIS WEEK

1. Health
2. Being
3. Being there
4. Love
5. Generosity
6. Serendipity

INHALE.EXHALE.REPEAT.

10/16 MON

Natasha

☐ AM YOGA ▨ PM YOGA ☐ MEDITATION

10/17 TUE

☐ AM YOGA ☐ PM YOGA ☐ MEDITATION

10/18 WED

☐ AM YOGA ☐ PM YOGA ☐ MEDITATION

10/19 THU

Pain Body Sign-up   Ok
("Shaking exercise")

☐ AM YOGA ☐ PM YOGA ▨ MEDITATION

INHALE. EXHALE. REPEAT.

OR

☐ AM YOGA ☐ PM YOGA ▨ MEDITATION

ASA 2017 - Chandler presented / Dr. Cote present
lost glasses in Uber a FOUND them
Scan T12 - Partial
Outlined plan for next week
Carolyn Myss : [OBSERVATION]

☐ AM YOGA ☐ PM YOGA ▨ MEDITATION

☐ AM YOGA ☐ PM YOGA ☐ MEDITATION

THINGS MOST GRATEFUL FOR THIS WEEK

GRATI TUDE

1.
2.
3.
4.
5.
6.

INHALE. EXHALE. REPEAT.

10/30 MON

Feeling great with respect to low back pain. But with change of seasons, my overall energy level is low. The fact I can focus on several writing deadlines is a good thing.

6:15 PM - Natasha's Class @ DUY — TWISTS

☐ AM YOGA ▨ PM YOGA ▨ MEDITATION

10/31 TUE

AM Meditation — Slow/prexuce/breakfast
Being in the moment throughout the day and accomplishing administrative tasks as they were presenting itself.
Delayed on Chapter writing for Sci. American
9PM YOGA → Slow Flow with Meghan

☐ AM YOGA ▨ PM YOGA ▨ MEDITATION

11/01 WED

Is this gap in personal practice telling me something?

Is all this work, endless work

☐ AM YOGA ☐ PM YOGA ☐ MEDITATION of meaningful purpose?

11/02 THU

Is this extreme work effort worth all the personal practice?
Is this work a 'personal' practice?
What does the emptiness brings?

SFN 2017 - Washington DC

☐ AM YOGA ☐ PM YOGA ☐ MEDITATION

INHALE.EXHALE.REPEAT.

Be the one with awareness
So that all / every thing about
personal self dissapears!
peter Cutler

11/03 FRI

☐ AM YOGA ☐ PM YOGA ☐ MEDITATION

"Ask Your body for Forgiveness.
It all starts here!"
_____ InstaPost 11/14/17

11/04 SAT

☐ AM YOGA ☐ PM YOGA ☐ MEDITATION

o Press Conference o SFN 2017 11/13/17
Truth — What is truth?
Truth is not Sensational!
Truth is most boring thing!
Truth is [?] LIFE [?]

11/05 SUN

☐ AM YOGA ☐ PM YOGA ☐ MEDITATION

THINGS MOST GRATEFUL FOR THIS WEEK

GRATITUDE

1. Being
2. Aware of Awareness
3. Being below a above the Clouds — Meditation
4. Being always there
5. Nothing is Good or Bad
6. Every Moment is Perfect

INHALE.EXHALE.REPEAT.

11/13 MON

SFN Conference — Washington DC

☐ Dynamic Poster

☑ Press Conference ——→ Featured in several articles

Momofuku Dinner
Lincoln Memorial, Vietnam Memorial

☐ AM YOGA ☐ PM YOGA ☑ MEDITATION

11/14 TUE

~~Flight~~
Meditation
Reading

" The balm of game changer requires global agency & imagination which begins with the unknown & takes into account our relational interdependency. It requires radical openness, a speculative attitude, pleasure in engaging with the unknown & a willingness to think beyond—

☐ AM YOGA ☐ PM YOGA ☑ MEDITATION

11/15 WED

Transporting all the remaining things from Serbia (valuables, furniture, china, gobelins)

Let yourself be silently drawn by the stronger pull of what you really love.

☐ AM YOGA ☐ PM YOGA ☐ MEDITATION

11/16 THU

☐ AM YOGA ☐ PM YOGA ☐ MEDITATION

INHALE. EXHALE. REPEAT.

2ND Call

11/17
FRI

☐ AM YOGA ☐ PM YOGA ▨ MEDITATION ⊙ work

11/18
SAT

Simply ~~embrace~~ *Accept* the moment as is &
Simply embrace the next moment with
Novelty, freshness, renewed energy, w/o any
judgements of what was or clinging to the past

⊙ kino yoga ⊙ Northend yoga #workshop

our current dimensions of time & space." *From Ecologies of

▨ AM YOGA ▨ PM YOGA ▨ MEDITATION Practice * @marisierra —

11/19
SUN

* Lean into the uncertainty with embodied presence *
Honor the eternal dance between known & unknown, ⎫ just
hope & despair, history & Futurism, beauty & chaos ⎬ words
                                                    ⎭ that
🎂 ROSIE's BIRTHDAY   ⊙ kino yoga #backbendspecial! are not
                             ⊙ Northend #backbendspecial
▨ AM YOGA ▨ PM YOGA ▨ MEDITATION   #workshop #ashtanga

THINGS MOST GRATEFUL FOR THIS WEEK

GRATI
TUDE

1. Health
2. Knowledge   HAVING NO PREFERENCES,
3. Glamour   THE WHOLE WORLD IS
4. Responsibility   A JOY #petercutler
5. Service,
6. abundance

INHALE. EXHALE. REPEAT.

11/20 MON

Fazed by nothing. Awed by at everything.
★ DAILY AFFIRMATIONS ★

- I trust that good things are comming my way
- I am abundant as fuck
- I choose to live for love
- Today, I am confident & Courageous

☐ AM YOGA ■ PM YOGA ☐ MEDITATION   Natasha's Class @DUY

11/21 TUE

- I find ease in my mind & body
- I love not giving a fuck.

Walking Meditation   @ cody app
☐ AM YOGA ■ PM YOGA ☐ MEDITATION Home Practice / Meghan Currie

WED

9AM - Meeting with a Chief
11-8 PM Shift OR (talk with Dr. Seefelder)

☐ AM YOGA ☐ PM YOGA ■ MEDITATION

THU

CLEANING DAY
TURKEY DAY
GRATITUDE DAY

☐ AM YOGA ☐ PM YOGA ☐ MEDITATION

INHALE. EXHALE. REPEAT.

Radiology Call

FRI

☐ AM YOGA ☐ PM YOGA ☒ MEDITATION *Walking Meditation*

Shopping with MAX

SAT

☐ AM YOGA ☐ PM YOGA ☒ MEDITATION

Basketball at BU
READING DAY

SUN

☐ AM YOGA ☐ PM YOGA ☒ MEDITATION

THINGS MOST GRATEFUL FOR THIS WEEK

GRATI TUDE

1. ABUNDANCE
2. SERVICE
3. Health
4. Beauty
5. Joy
6. Life Force

INHALE. EXHALE. REPEAT.

11/27/17
MON

* Chaturanga * CORE
• Spill palms back with
• Chest femucial
  UTKATASANA
  MALASANA
  BALASANA

6:15 PM Natasha's class

☐ AM YOGA ▦ PM YOGA ☐ MEDITATION

11/28/17
TUE

7:30 PM JoJo's Class

☐ AM YOGA ▦ PM YOGA ☐ MEDITATION

11/29
WED

☐ AM YOGA ☐ PM YOGA ☐ MEDITATION READING

11/30
THU

☐ AM YOGA ☐ PM YOGA ☐ MEDITATION

INHALE.EXHALE.REPEAT.

tms Course
#DANIEL BROWN PhD

12/1
FRI

☐ AM YOGA   ☐ PM YOGA   ▨ MEDITATION

tms Course
#DANIEL BROWN PhD

12/2
SAT

☐ AM YOGA   ☐ PM YOGA   ▨ MEDITATION

Reading: Brenée Brow "Nto Wilderness"
Reading a Practicing from KINO's BOOK
Ashtanga Yoga I
▨ Seating Sequences
. "PRACTICE EVERY DAY"

12/3
SUN

☐ AM YOGA   ▨ PM YOGA   ▨ MEDITATION

THINGS MOST GRATEFUL FOR THIS WEEK

GRATI TUDE

1. Beauty
2. Health
3. Abundance
4. Presence
5. Awakening
6. LOVE

INHALE.EXHALE.REPEAT.

FULL MOON

12/4
MON

X Late work

☐ AM YOGA ☐ PM YOGA ☐ MEDITATION

12/5
TUE

X Late work
Lecture by Allan Watts
Reading at Night

☐ AM YOGA ☐ PM YOGA ☐ MEDITATION

WED

☐ AM YOGA ☐ PM YOGA ☐ MEDITATION

THU

☐ AM YOGA ☐ PM YOGA ☐ MEDITATION

INHALE.EXHALE.REPEAT.

	FRI

- [ ] AM YOGA - [ ] PM YOGA - [ ] MEDITATION

	12/22/17
	SAT

SEEK: What you seek is already looking for you.
LIGHT: Bring LIGHT to each interaction
SOFTNESS: Notice the baseline softness beneath it all

- [ ] AM YOGA - [ ] PM YOGA - [ ] MEDITATION

	SUN

- [ ] AM YOGA - [ ] PM YOGA - [ ] MEDITATION

THINGS MOST GRATEFUL FOR THIS WEEK

	GRATI TUDE

1.
2.
3.
4.
5.
6.

INHALE.EXHALE.REPEAT.

MON

- [ ] AM YOGA
- [ ] PM YOGA
- [ ] MEDITATION

TUE

- [ ] AM YOGA
- [ ] PM YOGA
- [ ] MEDITATION

WED

- [ ] AM YOGA
- [ ] PM YOGA
- [ ] MEDITATION

THU

- [ ] AM YOGA
- [ ] PM YOGA
- [ ] MEDITATION

INHALE. EXHALE. REPEAT.

FRI

_____
_____
_____
_____
_____

☐ AM YOGA　☐ PM YOGA　☐ MEDITATION

SAT

_____
_____
_____
_____
_____

☐ AM YOGA　☐ PM YOGA　☐ MEDITATION

SUN

_____
_____
_____
_____
_____

☐ AM YOGA　☐ PM YOGA　☐ MEDITATION

THINGS MOST GRATEFUL FOR THIS WEEK

GRATITUDE

1.
2.
3.
4.
5.
6.

INHALE.EXHALE.REPEAT.

MON

- [ ] AM YOGA
- [ ] PM YOGA
- [ ] MEDITATION

TUE

- [ ] AM YOGA
- [ ] PM YOGA
- [ ] MEDITATION

WED

- [ ] AM YOGA
- [ ] PM YOGA
- [ ] MEDITATION

THU

- [ ] AM YOGA
- [ ] PM YOGA
- [ ] MEDITATION

INHALE.EXHALE.REPEAT.

FRI

_____
_____
_____
_____
_____
_____

☐ AM YOGA ☐ PM YOGA ☐ MEDITATION

SAT

_____
_____
_____
_____
_____
_____

☐ AM YOGA ☐ PM YOGA ☐ MEDITATION

SUN

_____
_____
_____
_____
_____
_____

☐ AM YOGA ☐ PM YOGA ☐ MEDITATION

THINGS MOST GRATEFUL FOR THIS WEEK

GRATITUDE

1.
2.
3.
4.
5.
6.

INHALE.EXHALE.REPEAT.

MON

_____
_____
_____
_____
_____
_____

☐ AM YOGA ☐ PM YOGA ☐ MEDITATION

TUE

_____
_____
_____
_____
_____
_____

☐ AM YOGA ☐ PM YOGA ☐ MEDITATION

WED

_____
_____
_____
_____
_____
_____

☐ AM YOGA ☐ PM YOGA ☐ MEDITATION

THU

_____
_____
_____
_____
_____
_____

☐ AM YOGA ☐ PM YOGA ☐ MEDITATION

INHALE. EXHALE. REPEAT.

FRI

_____
_____
_____
_____
_____
_____

☐ AM YOGA ☐ PM YOGA ☐ MEDITATION

SAT

_____
_____
_____
_____
_____
_____

☐ AM YOGA ☐ PM YOGA ☐ MEDITATION

SUN

_____
_____
_____
_____
_____
_____

☐ AM YOGA ☐ PM YOGA ☐ MEDITATION

THINGS MOST GRATEFUL FOR THIS WEEK

GRATITUDE

1. _____
2. _____
3. _____
4. _____
5. _____
6. _____

INHALE.EXHALE.REPEAT.

MON

_____

☐ AM YOGA ☐ PM YOGA ☐ MEDITATION

TUE

_____

☐ AM YOGA ☐ PM YOGA ☐ MEDITATION

WED

_____

☐ AM YOGA ☐ PM YOGA ☐ MEDITATION

THU

_____

☐ AM YOGA ☐ PM YOGA ☐ MEDITATION

INHALE. EXHALE. REPEAT.

_____
FRI

_____
_____
_____
_____
_____

☐ AM YOGA   ☐ PM YOGA   ☐ MEDITATION

_____
SAT

_____
_____
_____
_____
_____

☐ AM YOGA   ☐ PM YOGA   ☐ MEDITATION

_____
SUN

_____
_____
_____
_____
_____

☐ AM YOGA   ☐ PM YOGA   ☐ MEDITATION

THINGS MOST GRATEFUL FOR THIS WEEK
GRATI TUDE

1.
2.
3.
4.
5.
6.

INHALE.EXHALE.REPEAT.

MON
_____
_____
_____
_____
_____
_____

☐ AM YOGA   ☐ PM YOGA   ☐ MEDITATION

TUE
_____
_____
_____
_____
_____
_____

☐ AM YOGA   ☐ PM YOGA   ☐ MEDITATION

WED
_____
_____
_____
_____
_____
_____

☐ AM YOGA   ☐ PM YOGA   ☐ MEDITATION

THU
_____
_____
_____
_____
_____
_____

☐ AM YOGA   ☐ PM YOGA   ☐ MEDITATION

INHALE. EXHALE. REPEAT.

FRI

_____
_____
_____
_____
_____
_____

☐ AM YOGA ☐ PM YOGA ☐ MEDITATION

SAT

_____
_____
_____
_____
_____
_____

☐ AM YOGA ☐ PM YOGA ☐ MEDITATION

SUN

_____
_____
_____
_____
_____
_____

☐ AM YOGA ☐ PM YOGA ☐ MEDITATION

THINGS MOST GRATEFUL FOR THIS WEEK

GRATI TUDE

1. _____
2. _____
3. _____
4. _____
5. _____
6. _____

INHALE. EXHALE. REPEAT.

MON

☐ AM YOGA ☐ PM YOGA ☐ MEDITATION

TUE

☐ AM YOGA ☐ PM YOGA ☐ MEDITATION

WED

☐ AM YOGA ☐ PM YOGA ☐ MEDITATION

THU

☐ AM YOGA ☐ PM YOGA ☐ MEDITATION

INHALE.EXHALE.REPEAT.

FRI

_____
_____
_____
_____
_____
_____

☐ AM YOGA ☐ PM YOGA ☐ MEDITATION

SAT

_____
_____
_____
_____
_____
_____

☐ AM YOGA ☐ PM YOGA ☐ MEDITATION

SUN

_____
_____
_____
_____
_____
_____

☐ AM YOGA ☐ PM YOGA ☐ MEDITATION

THINGS MOST GRATEFUL FOR THIS WEEK

GRATITUDE

1.
2.
3.
4.
5.
6.

INHALE.EXHALE.REPEAT.

MON

☐ AM YOGA   ☐ PM YOGA   ☐ MEDITATION

TUE

☐ AM YOGA   ☐ PM YOGA   ☐ MEDITATION

WED

☐ AM YOGA   ☐ PM YOGA   ☐ MEDITATION

THU

☐ AM YOGA   ☐ PM YOGA   ☐ MEDITATION

INHALE. EXHALE. REPEAT.

FRI

_____

_____

_____

_____

☐ AM YOGA ☐ PM YOGA ☐ MEDITATION

SAT

_____

_____

_____

_____

☐ AM YOGA ☐ PM YOGA ☐ MEDITATION

SUN

_____

_____

_____

_____

☐ AM YOGA ☐ PM YOGA ☐ MEDITATION

THINGS MOST GRATEFUL FOR THIS WEEK

GRATITUDE

1. _____
2. _____
3. _____
4. _____
5. _____
6. _____

INHALE. EXHALE. REPEAT.

MON
_____
_____
_____
_____
_____
_____

☐ AM YOGA   ☐ PM YOGA   ☐ MEDITATION

TUE
_____
_____
_____
_____
_____
_____

☐ AM YOGA   ☐ PM YOGA   ☐ MEDITATION

WED
_____
_____
_____
_____
_____
_____

☐ AM YOGA   ☐ PM YOGA   ☐ MEDITATION

THU
_____
_____
_____
_____
_____

☐ AM YOGA   ☐ PM YOGA   ☐ MEDITATION

INHALE. EXHALE. REPEAT.

FRI

_____
_____
_____
_____
_____

☐ AM YOGA ☐ PM YOGA ☐ MEDITATION

SAT

_____
_____
_____
_____
_____

☐ AM YOGA ☐ PM YOGA ☐ MEDITATION

SUN

_____
_____
_____
_____
_____

☐ AM YOGA ☐ PM YOGA ☐ MEDITATION

THINGS MOST GRATEFUL FOR THIS WEEK

GRATITUDE

1. _____
2. _____
3. _____
4. _____
5. _____
6. _____

INHALE. EXHALE. REPEAT.

MON

_____
_____
_____
_____
_____
_____
_____

☐ AM YOGA ☐ PM YOGA ☐ MEDITATION

TUE

_____
_____
_____
_____
_____
_____
_____

☐ AM YOGA ☐ PM YOGA ☐ MEDITATION

WED

_____
_____
_____
_____
_____
_____
_____

☐ AM YOGA ☐ PM YOGA ☐ MEDITATION

THU

_____
_____
_____
_____
_____
_____
_____

☐ AM YOGA ☐ PM YOGA ☐ MEDITATION

INHALE.EXHALE.REPEAT.

FRI

_____

_____

_____

_____

_____

☐ AM YOGA   ☐ PM YOGA   ☐ MEDITATION

SAT

_____

_____

_____

_____

_____

☐ AM YOGA   ☐ PM YOGA   ☐ MEDITATION

SUN

_____

_____

_____

_____

_____

☐ AM YOGA   ☐ PM YOGA   ☐ MEDITATION

THINGS MOST GRATEFUL FOR THIS WEEK

GRATITUDE

1. _____
2. _____
3. _____
4. _____
5. _____
6. _____

INHALE.EXHALE.REPEAT.

MON

_____
_____
_____
_____
_____
_____

☐ AM YOGA   ☐ PM YOGA   ☐ MEDITATION

TUE

_____
_____
_____
_____
_____
_____

☐ AM YOGA   ☐ PM YOGA   ☐ MEDITATION

WED

_____
_____
_____
_____
_____
_____

☐ AM YOGA   ☐ PM YOGA   ☐ MEDITATION

THU

_____
_____
_____
_____
_____
_____

☐ AM YOGA   ☐ PM YOGA   ☐ MEDITATION

INHALE. EXHALE. REPEAT.

FRI

_____
_____
_____
_____
_____
_____

☐ AM YOGA ☐ PM YOGA ☐ MEDITATION

SAT

_____
_____
_____
_____
_____
_____

☐ AM YOGA ☐ PM YOGA ☐ MEDITATION

SUN

_____
_____
_____
_____
_____
_____

☐ AM YOGA ☐ PM YOGA ☐ MEDITATION

THINGS MOST GRATEFUL FOR THIS WEEK

GRATITUDE

1. _____
2. _____
3. _____
4. _____
5. _____
6. _____

INHALE.EXHALE.REPEAT.

MON

_____

☐ AM YOGA ☐ PM YOGA ☐ MEDITATION

TUE

_____

☐ AM YOGA ☐ PM YOGA ☐ MEDITATION

WED

_____

☐ AM YOGA ☐ PM YOGA ☐ MEDITATION

THU

_____

☐ AM YOGA ☐ PM YOGA ☐ MEDITATION

INHALE.EXHALE.REPEAT.

FRI

_____

☐ AM YOGA   ☐ PM YOGA   ☐ MEDITATION

SAT

_____

☐ AM YOGA   ☐ PM YOGA   ☐ MEDITATION

SUN

_____

☐ AM YOGA   ☐ PM YOGA   ☐ MEDITATION

THINGS MOST GRATEFUL FOR THIS WEEK

GRATITUDE

1.
2.
3.
4.
5.
6.

INHALE.EXHALE.REPEAT.

MON

☐ AM YOGA ☐ PM YOGA ☐ MEDITATION

TUE

☐ AM YOGA ☐ PM YOGA ☐ MEDITATION

WED

☐ AM YOGA ☐ PM YOGA ☐ MEDITATION

THU

☐ AM YOGA ☐ PM YOGA ☐ MEDITATION

INHALE. EXHALE. REPEAT.

FRI

_____

☐ AM YOGA   ☐ PM YOGA   ☐ MEDITATION

SAT

_____

☐ AM YOGA   ☐ PM YOGA   ☐ MEDITATION

SUN

_____

☐ AM YOGA   ☐ PM YOGA   ☐ MEDITATION

THINGS MOST GRATEFUL FOR THIS WEEK

GRATITUDE

1.
2.
3.
4.
5.
6.

INHALE. EXHALE. REPEAT.

MON

_____

☐ AM YOGA   ☐ PM YOGA   ☐ MEDITATION

TUE

_____

☐ AM YOGA   ☐ PM YOGA   ☐ MEDITATION

WED

_____

☐ AM YOGA   ☐ PM YOGA   ☐ MEDITATION

THU

_____

☐ AM YOGA   ☐ PM YOGA   ☐ MEDITATION

INHALE. EXHALE. REPEAT.

FRI

_____

☐ AM YOGA   ☐ PM YOGA   ☐ MEDITATION

SAT

_____

☐ AM YOGA   ☐ PM YOGA   ☐ MEDITATION

SUN

_____

☐ AM YOGA   ☐ PM YOGA   ☐ MEDITATION

THINGS MOST GRATEFUL FOR THIS WEEK

GRATITUDE

1.
2.
3.
4.
5.
6.

INHALE.EXHALE.REPEAT.

MON

_____
_____
_____
_____
_____
_____

☐ AM YOGA   ☐ PM YOGA   ☐ MEDITATION

TUE

_____
_____
_____
_____
_____
_____

☐ AM YOGA   ☐ PM YOGA   ☐ MEDITATION

WED

_____
_____
_____
_____
_____
_____

☐ AM YOGA   ☐ PM YOGA   ☐ MEDITATION

THU

_____
_____
_____
_____
_____

☐ AM YOGA   ☐ PM YOGA   ☐ MEDITATION

INHALE.EXHALE.REPEAT.

FRI

_____
_____
_____
_____
_____
_____

☐ AM YOGA   ☐ PM YOGA   ☐ MEDITATION

SAT

_____
_____
_____
_____
_____
_____

☐ AM YOGA   ☐ PM YOGA   ☐ MEDITATION

SUN

_____
_____
_____
_____
_____
_____

☐ AM YOGA   ☐ PM YOGA   ☐ MEDITATION

THINGS MOST GRATEFUL FOR THIS WEEK

GRATITUDE

1. _____
2. _____
3. _____
4. _____
5. _____
6. _____

INHALE. EXHALE. REPEAT.

MON

_____

☐ AM YOGA ☐ PM YOGA ☐ MEDITATION

TUE

_____

☐ AM YOGA ☐ PM YOGA ☐ MEDITATION

WED

_____

☐ AM YOGA ☐ PM YOGA ☐ MEDITATION

THU

_____

☐ AM YOGA ☐ PM YOGA ☐ MEDITATION

INHALE. EXHALE. REPEAT.

FRI

_____

_____

_____

_____

_____

☐ AM YOGA   ☐ PM YOGA   ☐ MEDITATION

SAT

_____

_____

_____

_____

_____

☐ AM YOGA   ☐ PM YOGA   ☐ MEDITATION

SUN

_____

_____

_____

_____

_____

☐ AM YOGA   ☐ PM YOGA   ☐ MEDITATION

THINGS MOST GRATEFUL FOR THIS WEEK

GRATITUDE

1. _____
2. _____
3. _____
4. _____
5. _____
6. _____

INHALE. EXHALE. REPEAT.

MON

_____

☐ AM YOGA ☐ PM YOGA ☐ MEDITATION

TUE

_____

☐ AM YOGA ☐ PM YOGA ☐ MEDITATION

WED

_____

☐ AM YOGA ☐ PM YOGA ☐ MEDITATION

THU

_____

☐ AM YOGA ☐ PM YOGA ☐ MEDITATION

INHALE. EXHALE. REPEAT.

FRI

_____

☐ AM YOGA ☐ PM YOGA ☐ MEDITATION

SAT

☐ AM YOGA ☐ PM YOGA ☐ MEDITATION

SUN

☐ AM YOGA ☐ PM YOGA ☐ MEDITATION

THINGS MOST GRATEFUL FOR THIS WEEK

GRATITUDE

1.
2.
3.
4.
5.
6.

INHALE.EXHALE.REPEAT.

MON

☐ AM YOGA ☐ PM YOGA ☐ MEDITATION

TUE

☐ AM YOGA ☐ PM YOGA ☐ MEDITATION

WED

☐ AM YOGA ☐ PM YOGA ☐ MEDITATION

THU

☐ AM YOGA ☐ PM YOGA ☐ MEDITATION

INHALE. EXHALE. REPEAT.

FRI

_____

_____

_____

_____

_____

_____

☐ AM YOGA   ☐ PM YOGA   ☐ MEDITATION

SAT

_____

_____

_____

_____

_____

_____

☐ AM YOGA   ☐ PM YOGA   ☐ MEDITATION

SUN

_____

_____

_____

_____

_____

_____

☐ AM YOGA   ☐ PM YOGA   ☐ MEDITATION

THINGS MOST GRATEFUL FOR THIS WEEK

GRATITUDE

1.
2.
3.
4.
5.
6.

INHALE. EXHALE. REPEAT.

MON

_____
_____
_____
_____
_____

☐ AM YOGA   ☐ PM YOGA   ☐ MEDITATION

TUE

_____
_____
_____
_____
_____

☐ AM YOGA   ☐ PM YOGA   ☐ MEDITATION

WED

_____
_____
_____
_____
_____

☐ AM YOGA   ☐ PM YOGA   ☐ MEDITATION

THU

_____
_____
_____
_____
_____

☐ AM YOGA   ☐ PM YOGA   ☐ MEDITATION

INHALE. EXHALE. REPEAT.

_____

	FRI

☐ AM YOGA ☐ PM YOGA ☐ MEDITATION

	SAT

☐ AM YOGA ☐ PM YOGA ☐ MEDITATION

	SUN

☐ AM YOGA ☐ PM YOGA ☐ MEDITATION

THINGS MOST GRATEFUL FOR THIS WEEK

GRATITUDE

1.
2.
3.
4.
5.
6.

INHALE. EXHALE. REPEAT.

MON

AM YOGA   PM YOGA   MEDITATION

TUE

AM YOGA   PM YOGA   MEDITATION

WED

AM YOGA   PM YOGA   MEDITATION

THU

AM YOGA   PM YOGA   MEDITATION

INHALE. EXHALE. REPEAT.

FRI

☐ AM YOGA ☐ PM YOGA ☐ MEDITATION

SAT

☐ AM YOGA ☐ PM YOGA ☐ MEDITATION

SUN

☐ AM YOGA ☐ PM YOGA ☐ MEDITATION

THINGS MOST GRATEFUL FOR THIS WEEK

GRATITUDE

1.
2.
3.
4.
5.
6.

INHALE.EXHALE.REPEAT.

MON

☐ AM YOGA ☐ PM YOGA ☐ MEDITATION

TUE

☐ AM YOGA ☐ PM YOGA ☐ MEDITATION

WED

☐ AM YOGA ☐ PM YOGA ☐ MEDITATION

THU

☐ AM YOGA ☐ PM YOGA ☐ MEDITATION

INHALE. EXHALE. REPEAT.

FRI

_____
_____
_____
_____
_____
_____

☐ AM YOGA ☐ PM YOGA ☐ MEDITATION

SAT

_____
_____
_____
_____
_____
_____

☐ AM YOGA ☐ PM YOGA ☐ MEDITATION

SUN

_____
_____
_____
_____
_____

☐ AM YOGA ☐ PM YOGA ☐ MEDITATION

THINGS MOST GRATEFUL FOR THIS WEEK

GRATITUDE

1. _____
2. _____
3. _____
4. _____
5. _____
6. _____

INHALE. EXHALE. REPEAT.

MON

_____

☐ AM YOGA   ☐ PM YOGA   ☐ MEDITATION

TUE

_____

☐ AM YOGA   ☐ PM YOGA   ☐ MEDITATION

WED

_____

☐ AM YOGA   ☐ PM YOGA   ☐ MEDITATION

THU

_____

☐ AM YOGA   ☐ PM YOGA   ☐ MEDITATION

INHALE. EXHALE. REPEAT.

_____
_____
_____
_____
_____
_____

FRI

☐ AM YOGA   ☐ PM YOGA   ☐ MEDITATION

_____
_____
_____
_____
_____
_____

SAT

☐ AM YOGA   ☐ PM YOGA   ☐ MEDITATION

_____
_____
_____
_____
_____
_____

SUN

☐ AM YOGA   ☐ PM YOGA   ☐ MEDITATION

THINGS MOST GRATEFUL FOR THIS WEEK

GRATITUDE

1. _____
2. _____
3. _____
4. _____
5. _____
6. _____

INHALE.EXHALE.REPEAT.

MON

_____

☐ AM YOGA ☐ PM YOGA ☐ MEDITATION

TUE

_____

☐ AM YOGA ☐ PM YOGA ☐ MEDITATION

WED

_____

☐ AM YOGA ☐ PM YOGA ☐ MEDITATION

THU

_____

☐ AM YOGA ☐ PM YOGA ☐ MEDITATION

INHALE. EXHALE. REPEAT.

FRI

☐ AM YOGA ☐ PM YOGA ☐ MEDITATION

SAT

☐ AM YOGA ☐ PM YOGA ☐ MEDITATION

SUN

☐ AM YOGA ☐ PM YOGA ☐ MEDITATION

THINGS MOST GRATEFUL FOR THIS WEEK

GRATITUDE

1.
2.
3.
4.
5.
6.

INHALE.EXHALE.REPEAT.

MON

_____
_____
_____
_____
_____

☐ AM YOGA ☐ PM YOGA ☐ MEDITATION

TUE

_____
_____
_____
_____
_____

☐ AM YOGA ☐ PM YOGA ☐ MEDITATION

WED

_____
_____
_____
_____
_____

☐ AM YOGA ☐ PM YOGA ☐ MEDITATION

THU

_____
_____
_____
_____
_____

☐ AM YOGA ☐ PM YOGA ☐ MEDITATION

INHALE. EXHALE. REPEAT.

FRI

_____
_____
_____
_____
_____
_____

☐ AM YOGA ☐ PM YOGA ☐ MEDITATION

SAT

_____
_____
_____
_____
_____
_____

☐ AM YOGA ☐ PM YOGA ☐ MEDITATION

SUN

_____
_____
_____
_____
_____
_____

☐ AM YOGA ☐ PM YOGA ☐ MEDITATION

THINGS MOST GRATEFUL FOR THIS WEEK

GRATITUDE

1.
2.
3.
4.
5.
6.

INHALE.EXHALE.REPEAT.

MON

☐ AM YOGA   ☐ PM YOGA   ☐ MEDITATION

TUE

☐ AM YOGA   ☐ PM YOGA   ☐ MEDITATION

WED

☐ AM YOGA   ☐ PM YOGA   ☐ MEDITATION

THU

☐ AM YOGA   ☐ PM YOGA   ☐ MEDITATION

INHALE. EXHALE. REPEAT.

FRI

_____
_____
_____
_____
_____
_____
_____

☐ AM YOGA   ☐ PM YOGA   ☐ MEDITATION

SAT

_____
_____
_____
_____
_____
_____
_____

☐ AM YOGA   ☐ PM YOGA   ☐ MEDITATION

SUN

_____
_____
_____
_____
_____
_____

☐ AM YOGA   ☐ PM YOGA   ☐ MEDITATION

THINGS MOST GRATEFUL FOR THIS WEEK

GRATITUDE

1.
2.
3.
4.
5.
6.

INHALE.EXHALE.REPEAT.

MON

_____
_____
_____
_____
_____
_____

☐ AM YOGA   ☐ PM YOGA   ☐ MEDITATION

TUE

_____
_____
_____
_____
_____
_____

☐ AM YOGA   ☐ PM YOGA   ☐ MEDITATION

WED

_____
_____
_____
_____
_____
_____

☐ AM YOGA   ☐ PM YOGA   ☐ MEDITATION

THU

_____
_____
_____
_____
_____
_____

☐ AM YOGA   ☐ PM YOGA   ☐ MEDITATION

INHALE. EXHALE. REPEAT.

FRI

_____

_____

_____

_____

_____

_____

☐ AM YOGA   ☐ PM YOGA   ☐ MEDITATION

SAT

_____

_____

_____

_____

_____

_____

☐ AM YOGA   ☐ PM YOGA   ☐ MEDITATION

SUN

_____

_____

_____

_____

_____

_____

☐ AM YOGA   ☐ PM YOGA   ☐ MEDITATION

THINGS MOST GRATEFUL FOR THIS WEEK

GRATITUDE

1. _____
2. _____
3. _____
4. _____
5. _____
6. _____

INHALE. EXHALE. REPEAT.

MON

☐ AM YOGA　　☐ PM YOGA　　☐ MEDITATION

TUE

☐ AM YOGA　　☐ PM YOGA　　☐ MEDITATION

WED

☐ AM YOGA　　☐ PM YOGA　　☐ MEDITATION

THU

☐ AM YOGA　　☐ PM YOGA　　☐ MEDITATION

INHALE. EXHALE. REPEAT.

FRI

_____

☐ AM YOGA　☐ PM YOGA　☐ MEDITATION

SAT

_____

☐ AM YOGA　☐ PM YOGA　☐ MEDITATION

SUN

_____

☐ AM YOGA　☐ PM YOGA　☐ MEDITATION

THINGS MOST GRATEFUL FOR THIS WEEK

GRATITUDE

1.
2.
3.
4.
5.
6.

INHALE. EXHALE. REPEAT.

MON

_____
_____
_____
_____
_____

☐ AM YOGA ☐ PM YOGA ☐ MEDITATION

TUE

_____
_____
_____
_____
_____

☐ AM YOGA ☐ PM YOGA ☐ MEDITATION

WED

_____
_____
_____
_____
_____

☐ AM YOGA ☐ PM YOGA ☐ MEDITATION

THU

_____
_____
_____
_____
_____

☐ AM YOGA ☐ PM YOGA ☐ MEDITATION

INHALE. EXHALE. REPEAT.

FRI

_____

_____

_____

_____

_____

_____

☐ AM YOGA ☐ PM YOGA ☐ MEDITATION

SAT

_____

_____

_____

_____

_____

_____

☐ AM YOGA ☐ PM YOGA ☐ MEDITATION

SUN

_____

_____

_____

_____

_____

_____

☐ AM YOGA ☐ PM YOGA ☐ MEDITATION

THINGS MOST GRATEFUL FOR THIS WEEK

GRATITUDE

1.

2.

3.

4.

5.

6.

INHALE. EXHALE. REPEAT.

MON

☐ AM YOGA   ☐ PM YOGA   ☐ MEDITATION

TUE

☐ AM YOGA   ☐ PM YOGA   ☐ MEDITATION

WED

☐ AM YOGA   ☐ PM YOGA   ☐ MEDITATION

THU

☐ AM YOGA   ☐ PM YOGA   ☐ MEDITATION

INHALE. EXHALE. REPEAT.

_____

FRI

_____
_____
_____
_____
_____

☐ AM YOGA   ☐ PM YOGA   ☐ MEDITATION

_____

SAT

_____
_____
_____
_____
_____

☐ AM YOGA   ☐ PM YOGA   ☐ MEDITATION

_____

SUN

_____
_____
_____
_____
_____

☐ AM YOGA   ☐ PM YOGA   ☐ MEDITATION

THINGS MOST GRATEFUL FOR THIS WEEK

GRATITUDE

1.
2.
3.
4.
5.
6.

INHALE. EXHALE. REPEAT.

MON

☐ AM YOGA　　☐ PM YOGA　　☐ MEDITATION

TUE

☐ AM YOGA　　☐ PM YOGA　　☐ MEDITATION

WED

☐ AM YOGA　　☐ PM YOGA　　☐ MEDITATION

THU

☐ AM YOGA　　☐ PM YOGA　　☐ MEDITATION

INHALE.EXHALE.REPEAT.

FRI

_____

☐ AM YOGA   ☐ PM YOGA   ☐ MEDITATION

SAT

_____

☐ AM YOGA   ☐ PM YOGA   ☐ MEDITATION

SUN

_____

☐ AM YOGA   ☐ PM YOGA   ☐ MEDITATION

GRATITUDE

THINGS MOST GRATEFUL FOR THIS WEEK

1.
2.
3.
4.
5.
6.

INHALE. EXHALE. REPEAT.

MON

☐ AM YOGA   ☐ PM YOGA   ☐ MEDITATION

TUE

☐ AM YOGA   ☐ PM YOGA   ☐ MEDITATION

WED

☐ AM YOGA   ☐ PM YOGA   ☐ MEDITATION

THU

☐ AM YOGA   ☐ PM YOGA   ☐ MEDITATION

INHALE. EXHALE. REPEAT.

FRI

_____
_____
_____
_____
_____
_____

☐ AM YOGA   ☐ PM YOGA   ☐ MEDITATION

SAT

_____
_____
_____
_____
_____
_____

☐ AM YOGA   ☐ PM YOGA   ☐ MEDITATION

SUN

_____
_____
_____
_____
_____

☐ AM YOGA   ☐ PM YOGA   ☐ MEDITATION

THINGS MOST GRATEFUL FOR THIS WEEK

GRATITUDE

1. _____
2. _____
3. _____
4. _____
5. _____
6. _____

INHALE.EXHALE.REPEAT.

MON

☐ AM YOGA   ☐ PM YOGA   ☐ MEDITATION

TUE

☐ AM YOGA   ☐ PM YOGA   ☐ MEDITATION

WED

☐ AM YOGA   ☐ PM YOGA   ☐ MEDITATION

THU

☐ AM YOGA   ☐ PM YOGA   ☐ MEDITATION

INHALE. EXHALE. REPEAT.

FRI

_____
_____
_____
_____
_____
_____

☐ AM YOGA ☐ PM YOGA ☐ MEDITATION

SAT

_____
_____
_____
_____
_____
_____

☐ AM YOGA ☐ PM YOGA ☐ MEDITATION

SUN

_____
_____
_____
_____
_____
_____

☐ AM YOGA ☐ PM YOGA ☐ MEDITATION

THINGS MOST GRATEFUL FOR THIS WEEK

GRATITUDE

1. _____
2. _____
3. _____
4. _____
5. _____
6. _____

INHALE. EXHALE. REPEAT.

MON

☐ AM YOGA ☐ PM YOGA ☐ MEDITATION

TUE

☐ AM YOGA ☐ PM YOGA ☐ MEDITATION

WED

☐ AM YOGA ☐ PM YOGA ☐ MEDITATION

THU

☐ AM YOGA ☐ PM YOGA ☐ MEDITATION

INHALE. EXHALE. REPEAT.

FRI

_____

☐ AM YOGA   ☐ PM YOGA   ☐ MEDITATION

SAT

_____

☐ AM YOGA   ☐ PM YOGA   ☐ MEDITATION

SUN

_____

☐ AM YOGA   ☐ PM YOGA   ☐ MEDITATION

THINGS MOST GRATEFUL FOR THIS WEEK

GRATITUDE

1.
2.
3.
4.
5.
6.

INHALE. EXHALE. REPEAT.

MON

_____

☐ AM YOGA ☐ PM YOGA ☐ MEDITATION

TUE

_____

☐ AM YOGA ☐ PM YOGA ☐ MEDITATION

WED

_____

☐ AM YOGA ☐ PM YOGA ☐ MEDITATION

THU

_____

☐ AM YOGA ☐ PM YOGA ☐ MEDITATION

INHALE. EXHALE. REPEAT.

FRI

_____
_____
_____
_____
_____
_____

☐ AM YOGA   ☐ PM YOGA   ☐ MEDITATION

SAT

_____
_____
_____
_____
_____
_____

☐ AM YOGA   ☐ PM YOGA   ☐ MEDITATION

SUN

_____
_____
_____
_____
_____
_____

☐ AM YOGA   ☐ PM YOGA   ☐ MEDITATION

THINGS MOST GRATEFUL FOR THIS WEEK

GRATI TUDE

1. _____
2. _____
3. _____
4. _____
5. _____
6. _____

INHALE. EXHALE. REPEAT.

MON

☐ AM YOGA   ☐ PM YOGA   ☐ MEDITATION

TUE

☐ AM YOGA   ☐ PM YOGA   ☐ MEDITATION

WED

☐ AM YOGA   ☐ PM YOGA   ☐ MEDITATION

THU

☐ AM YOGA   ☐ PM YOGA   ☐ MEDITATION

INHALE. EXHALE. REPEAT.

	FRI

☐ AM YOGA ☐ PM YOGA ☐ MEDITATION

	SAT

☐ AM YOGA ☐ PM YOGA ☐ MEDITATION

	SUN

☐ AM YOGA ☐ PM YOGA ☐ MEDITATION

THINGS MOST GRATEFUL FOR THIS WEEK

	GRATI TUDE

1.
2.
3.
4.
5.
6.

INHALE.EXHALE.REPEAT.

MON

☐ AM YOGA ☐ PM YOGA ☐ MEDITATION

TUE

☐ AM YOGA ☐ PM YOGA ☐ MEDITATION

WED

☐ AM YOGA ☐ PM YOGA ☐ MEDITATION

THU

☐ AM YOGA ☐ PM YOGA ☐ MEDITATION

INHALE. EXHALE. REPEAT.

<table>
<tr><td></td><td>FRI</td></tr>
</table>

☐ AM YOGA   ☐ PM YOGA   ☐ MEDITATION

| | SAT |

☐ AM YOGA   ☐ PM YOGA   ☐ MEDITATION

| | SUN |

☐ AM YOGA   ☐ PM YOGA   ☐ MEDITATION

THINGS MOST GRATEFUL FOR THIS WEEK

GRATITUDE

1.
2.
3.
4.
5.
6.

INHALE. EXHALE. REPEAT.

MON

☐ AM YOGA   ☐ PM YOGA   ☐ MEDITATION

TUE

☐ AM YOGA   ☐ PM YOGA   ☐ MEDITATION

WED

☐ AM YOGA   ☐ PM YOGA   ☐ MEDITATION

THU

☐ AM YOGA   ☐ PM YOGA   ☐ MEDITATION

INHALE. EXHALE. REPEAT.

_____

FRI

_____
_____
_____
_____
_____
_____

☐ AM YOGA   ☐ PM YOGA   ☐ MEDITATION

_____

SAT

_____
_____
_____
_____
_____
_____

☐ AM YOGA   ☐ PM YOGA   ☐ MEDITATION

_____

SUN

_____
_____
_____
_____
_____
_____

☐ AM YOGA   ☐ PM YOGA   ☐ MEDITATION

THINGS MOST GRATEFUL FOR THIS WEEK

GRATITUDE

1. _____
2. _____
3. _____
4. _____
5. _____
6. _____

INHALE. EXHALE. REPEAT.

MON

_____

☐ AM YOGA ☐ PM YOGA ☐ MEDITATION

TUE

_____

☐ AM YOGA ☐ PM YOGA ☐ MEDITATION

WED

_____

☐ AM YOGA ☐ PM YOGA ☐ MEDITATION

THU

_____

☐ AM YOGA ☐ PM YOGA ☐ MEDITATION

INHALE. EXHALE. REPEAT.

FRI

_____

_____

_____

_____

_____

_____

☐ AM YOGA   ☐ PM YOGA   ☐ MEDITATION

SAT

_____

_____

_____

_____

_____

_____

☐ AM YOGA   ☐ PM YOGA   ☐ MEDITATION

SUN

_____

_____

_____

_____

_____

_____

☐ AM YOGA   ☐ PM YOGA   ☐ MEDITATION

THINGS MOST GRATEFUL FOR THIS WEEK

GRATITUDE

1.

2.

3.

4.

5.

6.

INHALE.EXHALE.REPEAT.

MON

☐ AM YOGA ☐ PM YOGA ☐ MEDITATION

TUE

☐ AM YOGA ☐ PM YOGA ☐ MEDITATION

WED

☐ AM YOGA ☐ PM YOGA ☐ MEDITATION

THU

☐ AM YOGA ☐ PM YOGA ☐ MEDITATION

INHALE. EXHALE. REPEAT.

FRI

_____
_____
_____
_____
_____
_____

☐ AM YOGA   ☐ PM YOGA   ☐ MEDITATION

SAT

_____
_____
_____
_____
_____
_____

☐ AM YOGA   ☐ PM YOGA   ☐ MEDITATION

SUN

_____
_____
_____
_____
_____

☐ AM YOGA   ☐ PM YOGA   ☐ MEDITATION

THINGS MOST GRATEFUL FOR THIS WEEK

GRATITUDE

1. _____
2. _____
3. _____
4. _____
5. _____
6. _____

INHALE.EXHALE.REPEAT.

MON

_____
_____
_____
_____
_____
_____

☐ AM YOGA   ☐ PM YOGA   ☐ MEDITATION

TUE

_____
_____
_____
_____
_____
_____

☐ AM YOGA   ☐ PM YOGA   ☐ MEDITATION

WED

_____
_____
_____
_____
_____
_____

☐ AM YOGA   ☐ PM YOGA   ☐ MEDITATION

THU

_____
_____
_____
_____
_____
_____

☐ AM YOGA   ☐ PM YOGA   ☐ MEDITATION

INHALE. EXHALE. REPEAT.

FRI

_____

☐ AM YOGA   ☐ PM YOGA   ☐ MEDITATION

SAT

_____

☐ AM YOGA   ☐ PM YOGA   ☐ MEDITATION

SUN

_____

☐ AM YOGA   ☐ PM YOGA   ☐ MEDITATION

THINGS MOST GRATEFUL FOR THIS WEEK

GRATI
TUDE

1.
2.
3.
4.
5.
6.

INHALE. EXHALE. REPEAT.

MON

☐ AM YOGA ☐ PM YOGA ☐ MEDITATION

TUE

☐ AM YOGA ☐ PM YOGA ☐ MEDITATION

WED

☐ AM YOGA ☐ PM YOGA ☐ MEDITATION

THU

☐ AM YOGA ☐ PM YOGA ☐ MEDITATION

INHALE. EXHALE. REPEAT.

FRI

_____

_____

_____

_____

_____

_____

☐ AM YOGA   ☐ PM YOGA   ☐ MEDITATION

SAT

_____

_____

_____

_____

_____

_____

☐ AM YOGA   ☐ PM YOGA   ☐ MEDITATION

SUN

_____

_____

_____

_____

_____

_____

☐ AM YOGA   ☐ PM YOGA   ☐ MEDITATION

THINGS MOST GRATEFUL FOR THIS WEEK

GRATITUDE

1.

2.

3.

4.

5.

6.

Made in the USA
Middletown, DE
04 September 2017